Womb with a View

Tales from the Delivery, Emergency and Operating Rooms

Dr. Rebecca Levy-Gantt

Womb with a View:
Tales from the Delivery, Emergency and Operating Rooms

© 2020 by Dr. Rebecca Levy-Gantt

ISBN: 978-1-941066-41-6

Book design by Jo-Anne Rosen

Cover design by Heather Belt

Wordrunner Press
Petaluma, California

Contents

Womb with a View

Preface

When I was young I wanted to be a writer. I wrote about field trips and baseball games for school newspapers in middle and high school and fictional stories for creative writing magazines in college. I thrived on writing and reporting different kinds of stories, but discovered what I liked most was reporting my own life experiences. Later, after several career changes, teacher, health counselor, physical therapist, I decided to become a physician — eventually specializing in obstetrics and gynecology. Each day in this field was filled with events and stories I recorded in my mind and wanted to share. The stories flowed and stirred an array of emotions. The life and work of this specialty is filled with the happy, sad, interesting, devastating, and unbelievable, sometimes all on the same day. These are the stories, all true, some composites, that have influenced and affected me. My hope is that they will resonate with your experiences. This is my labor of love, my life as an ObGyn.

1

This Ain't No Appendix! There's a Human in There!

I was perpetually exhausted and a bit dazed as a third-year medical student. The weeks were difficult. I was hardly getting any sleep. I was learning and, probably for the first time, started considering whether obstetrics and gynecology might be the specialty for me. This wasn't something I was consciously making a decision about — I was finding myself interested in everything going on. I was watching how exams were done. I was doing them on my own. I was voluntarily and without prodding looking up answers to questions patients were asking me. The whole reproductive system throughout all the different stages of a woman's life was fascinating. I was finally able to venture into that scary place one evening, the Labor and Delivery ward. I would be allowed to scrub in on what was going to take place in the OR.

This procedure started like any other: the usual ritual of scrubbing my hands and arms with antiseptic, slowly and completely; gowning; putting on gloves correctly so the sterile part of the glove never touched an unsterile part of my skin; staying out of everyone's way; not touching anything blue, which were the sterile drapes; and repeating my name and my piddly credentials to the OR staff. All present in the OR had to be documented for all procedures all the time.

I stood at my place at the operating table, doing my usual job — retractor-holding and watching the resident meticulously carve through the layers of the abdomen. Dr. B asked me to identify the peritoneum, the fascia, the bladder, the muscles, and blood vessels, making sure the right instrument was used for each layer, listing each part of the anatomy in the correct order.

This was suddenly not like any surgery I had seen. Dr. B reached a hand into this woman's uterus and out came a living, moving, crying little person. She was pulling out an actual baby from inside this small opening in the woman's belly.

I was mesmerized. The procedure had started out like so many operations I had witnessed, from near and far in many operating rooms since my first exposure as a medical student. I had observed. I had witnessed. I had occasionally even touched a patient that was having surgery. All of those operations had been somewhat similar. About four minutes into *this* surgery, we took a completely new direction. This was not an appendix, a gallbladder, or even an ovary or tumor. I was watching a living human being, being brought out into the world, kicking and screaming, covered in cheesy vernix and amniotic fluid, emerging from a sac that had been home for the past nine months. This, I thought, was pretty freaking amazing.

I tried not to show my feeling, which was "Why is everyone in this room not saying, 'Oh My God, this is amazing!'" I realized that no one acted like this was amazing because here babies were an everyday event, at every hour of the day and night, especially at night when everyone would have rather been asleep. Some of the residents didn't want to be doing deliveries at all. They would have rather been orthopedic surgeons or anesthesiologists. All *I* could think about during that first C section and for a long time after, was "How lucky these people are. They actually get to see all this and participate in these events every day. *I* want to do this! Wow. Just wow."

2

The Light Bulb Goes On

My rotation in ObGyn as a third year medical student lasted six weeks: hardly enough time to learn everything, but in a busy county hospital in Brooklyn, definitely enough time to see a variety of medical procedures. As I became familiar with the goings-on in Labor and Delivery, and was staying longer hours, and every third night overnight, I became friendly with many of the non-physician staff. I enjoyed talking with the nurses, the physician's assistants, and the midwives. The midwives were caring for patients and delivering babies very differently than the residents did. They seemed to form more of a sisterhood with each other and with the patients. Women supporting other women through their labors and deliveries was more a celebration than a job.

Residents were on a time clock, giving medication on schedule, urging stronger contractions, saying things like, "You're here to deliver" as if these women were machines and could push out a baby on cue. Midwives, on the other hand, waited long hours with laboring women, and were patient as long as nothing became worrisome. Each one of their

2 The Light Bulb Goes On

delivery notes, however, had to be inspected and signed off by a resident. If one of their deliveries became emergent, or in need of intervention, the residents were required to step in and take over — usually resulting in operative deliveries, meaning forceps, vacuum deliveries or unexpected C sections. The residents and midwives had a cordial but at times suspicious relationship. Residents seemed to love having midwives there to do deliveries, but hated having more work to do when a midwife delivery had to be transferred over. I asked if I could observe and participate in the midwife deliveries. The residents told me, "Of course, as long as you do the paperwork!" They were probably impressed with my lengthy, informational notes on the normal postpartum patients.

I observed, lurked, and stalked the midwife deliveries, learning about the different stages of labor and the natural interventions the midwives had at their fingertips to make patients feel better and calmer in labor. These deliveries were very different from some of the other deliveries I had seen, with screaming, bright lights and blood everywhere.

After observing a few deliveries from the far side of the delivery room, I was beginning to sense the pattern that would occur. Early on, things were calm. Patients would sleep or read, or even eat and walk around. Then things would get intense and loud. Pushing would sometimes go on for hours, and at the moment the delivery was imminent, a flurry of activity would occur to get everything ready. During one of my observations, the flurry started to happen, and the midwife said to me, "Come on over here and put on the gown and gloves."

I wondered if this was my invitation to the sisterhood. I did as I was told, and she pushed the rolling stool over to the edge of the bed where the birth was about to occur. She told me to sit down and I did. She was beside me, still encouraging the woman to push-2-3-4-5, using each contraction to gently ease the baby down the birth canal. When the head, with a full head of brown hair presented itself, the midwife gently put her hands over mine, and helped me to guide the baby's head out without allowing any tearing of the stretching tissues surrounding the baby. We performed the maneuvers of delivery, bringing the baby into the world, head, then shoulder, other shoulder, thorax, body, legs and feet. I placed the baby, umbilical cord still attached, on the mother's abdomen.

At that moment, something happened. This is still difficult to describe, but I know something profound happened. I felt it in every part of my being. I was not a religious person, not even particularly spiritual. When I lifted that baby, crying and slippery, onto his mom's belly, I felt something, some sort of energy. The proverbial light bulb went on. This is what I was called to do, my calling, my life's work. I was not deciding... This specialty had chosen me.

3

Is There a Doctor in the House? (Is It Me?)

A first year resident was on short call from 7 in the morning until 11 at night. When the night shift came on, the first year resident's responsibility was to know everything that was going on in the delivery room, to deal with all postpartum problems, to take all phone calls from the post-op gynecology floor for surgical patients, and to do all the vaginal deliveries that occurred on that shift with less and less supervision as time went on. A first year resident would also be the second assist on C sections since most C sections were the second year resident's job, assisted by the fourth year resident, who was actually teaching and guiding the more junior resident in performing the operation. An attending physician was also usually present. The attending was the doctor who had finished residency years earlier and was now in charge of supervising all residents. The attending would be close by but not involved in the hands-on aspect of the surgery unless there was a major complication.

One evening on call, I was paired with a busy second year resident, and the fourth year resident, Dr. C. The second year resident had been called down to the ER to see a gynecology patient, as was part of her on call responsibility. I was in the delivery room when one of the patients who had been laboring all day was declared a failure to progress. She had been having strong, regular contractions for several hours, yet her cervix was not changing. She was not going to achieve a vaginal delivery. We sometimes waited for hours. As long as progress was being made toward a vaginal delivery, we would continue to wait. Progress would sometimes come to a halt and no amount of waiting or medication was going to achieve that delivery.

I did what I would normally do in these cases — present her. That meant reporting the history of the patient along with all pertinent information to Dr. C, the fourth year resident, chronologically explaining in detail the circumstances of the patient's labor, and why I thought her situation warranted a C section. This was not an emergency, and after some discussion, Dr. C agreed with me. My job was then to discuss the C section with the patient, Ms. R, explain the situation, obtain her written consent, and write all the orders needed to get the C section started. I had to call the second year resident, so she would come to the delivery room to operate.

Within 15 minutes, the OR was ready, buzzing with personnel: the surgical tech, the pediatric nurse, a labor nurse, several students, the anesthesiologist, and me. The patient was wheeled in, and Dr. C and I were scrubbed and ready. Then from the outer corridor, one of the nurses called in to us and said the second year resident was stuck in the emergency room. A second patient just came in and had to be seen. Dr. C said, "No problem. We'll do it." I took that to mean that *she* would be the surgeon, and I would assist her. No one said anything different.

Ms. R's abdomen was prepped with a Betadine wash. Her entire body was covered with a sterile blue drape so the only area showing was the area where the incision was to be made. The scrub tech was ready. We were all standing at the patient's side. When Dr. C called "Scalpel," requesting the first instrument, I was shocked to see the tech handing it across the table in *my* direction. I was so shocked that I actually turned around to look behind me to see if she was really trying to hand the scalpel to me. Dr. C said, "Yes you! You've seen enough C sections. You should be able to do one by now!"

I immediately became incredibly nervous, but there was no time to think. There I was with a knife in my hand. Over the next 45 minutes, Dr. C proceeded to guide me, patiently but sometimes not-so-patiently, through all the many layers of the abdomen. She expected me to know, and then to recite, the layers in order — the skin, the subcuticular layer, the fascia, the rectus muscles and the peritoneum, then the uterus. She showed me how to place my right hand deep into the pelvis, into the uterus and under the head so the baby could be gently lifted upward and delivered. She had me call for my instruments, in the proper order, name the anatomy, order the correct medications, and decide which sutures to use, until we finally put together all the layers we had opened on the way in.

I had no time to stop and think about what I was doing or how I felt. The idea was to be comfortable doing every part of this procedure, to make it routine. Inside I felt anything but routine. I was happy and anxious and scared and exhilarated, but careful not to display any emotion. The entire experience was difficult and exhausting and confirmed what I already knew: this is the work I wanted to do.

Toward the end of the surgery, the second year resident returned from the ER, obviously glad the C section went on in her absence and almost too happy to tell me, "You did the surgery. Now *you* can do the dictation, and *you* can write the orders." The clock said 11:20 PM. I couldn't leave until all was done. Even though a new team was already in to take over, no one would do someone else's work. I didn't care. I was floating. I floated all the way home, way past midnight.

4

The Best Medicine

I was a first year resident on call on a weekend, where we did 24 hour shifts. Early on a Friday evening shift, Dr. M, the fourth year resident would sometimes make the rounds, walking through the post-surgical ward to make sure everything was quiet and nothing was brewing. He didn't have to, since if there was a question, a patient with a fever, or a medication to be ordered, I would have been the one called. Dr. M was doing this because he was concerned and cared about patients recovering from surgery. He wanted to make sure they were well taken care of or as he said, "Tucked in for the night." I thought how I could be tucking in my one-year-old and three-year-old, but this was my job.

One night shortly after 11, Dr. M told me to come walk around the wards with him to check on the patients. I followed, carrying my trusty notepad. We went into the rooms that included women who had had emergency C sections, a patient who had received a blood transfusion after a particularly long surgery, and others who had been admitted for various problems over the last few days. We visited Ms.

T's room, a mid-fifties woman who appeared critically ill. She was thin and frail, with bony facial features, and large patches where we could see her scalp through thinning hair. When we approached the room, it was dark. She was quiet although obviously awake. When I got closer, I saw she had several tubes and lines attached to her, and a drain coming out of who-knows-where, with fluid coming out of it. Dr. M approached Ms. T. Despite her weakness, she was obviously happy to see him. They chatted for a few minutes. He checked some numbers on her bedside chart and noted she had lost a lot of weight. Ms. T told him she was having trouble eating.

When we left her room, Dr. M said, "Come with me." I tried not to think about the most obvious thing that popped into my head: He was my boss, I had heard an occasional inappropriate comment from him; I didn't know him. Did I give him the wrong impression? Is he making a pass at me?

I did what he said. He was the fourth year resident, and I was a nobody. I did not expect that directive to entail following him down the corridor, past the double doors, through the lobby, and straight out of the hospital. First year residents were not allowed to be off site when on call, but yet here he was, pretty much ordering me to go with him, in violation of all the rules. My curiosity and apprehension increased when he got in his car in the doctors' parking lot and motioned me to get in. I cautiously complied, wondering, "What the hell is going on? Where are we going? Is this what he does every night?"

In the car, he told me he had seen Ms. T several times on his oncology rotation. Her cancer was quite advanced. As we spoke, the drive became more intriguing when we approached a nearby ice cream shop. Though this was New York, and it was not unusual to find an ice cream shop open after midnight, our visit was certainly anything but usual. Dr. M purchased a large chocolate milkshake, and we drove back to the hospital. All I kept thinking was, "Who leaves the hospital in the middle of the night? Why is he taking me with him? How much trouble would I be in if my beeper goes off for a major emergency?" Thankfully, the beeper didn't make a sound.

He had bought what appeared to be a mouthwatering milkshake but not taken a sip. At the hospital, we walked back to Ms. T's room, and Dr. M handed her the milkshake. She looked at him with what seemed like a combination of disbelief and gratitude, but she reached out weakly and took it. She took a small sip. Her eyes filled with tears, and so did mine. This was her *doctor,* who had made a very special trip, just for her, in the hope that her ailing body could tolerate this tasty treat and that she would feel a bit better.

At that moment, I witnessed how being a good doctor entailed much more than simply knowledge and technical skill. I saw how it is also about connecting in real time with real people, offering them kindness in addition to medical care. I thought, "Wow, imagine, this is just something that your doctor *does*!" I was a bit in awe and a bit confused but I decided at that moment whenever possible, *that* is how I wanted to make *my* patients feel someday. Dr. M didn't discuss interacting with patients with me as he generally didn't talk much. What he modeled through his actions made a huge impact on me and on my thoughts about what actually *could* be the norm for patient care. I knew the Hippocratic Oath said to do no harm, but to that I now added the Milkshake Oath: Be sure to make patients feel seen, respected, and cared for, and sometimes a milkshake may be just what the doctor ordered.

5

Two Tiny Feet

Obstetrics and gynecology is The Happy Specialty. Bringing life into the world is one of the best feelings and brings the most joy. Every woman remembers her delivery, not so much her gallbladder surgery or the surgeon. The happiness that comes with this field can be amazing. The sadness is truly heartbreaking. When things go wrong in obstetrics, they often go horribly wrong, unexpectedly wrong, and can result in damage and death to the mother and the baby, and leave deep emotional scars on family, friends, and health care providers.

A young woman, maybe in her early 20s, arrived one night during my first year night-call rotation. Ms. Z was about 22 weeks pregnant. She walked into the triage area of the delivery room. I was the point of first contact. Since pregnancies are counted in weeks, and a full-term pregnancy is 38 weeks, Ms. Z was a little over halfway there, about five and a half months pregnant.

By now, I had enough "experience" (always in quotations, because no first year resident has enough experience, just varying degrees of ignorance) to note details about any patient just upon their presentation, as to how emergent their situation was. Ms. Z *walked* in, which was good. She was not uncomfortable or symptomatic enough to have called an ambulance or be wheelchaired in or rolled in on a gurney. This was the night shift, which was a negative, because problems that are not truly emergencies can usually wait until morning. Patients who decide to go to the hospital after midnight usually at least *think* their situation is emergent.

Ms. Z was not making noise, no moaning, screaming, or crying, all good because that usually means she has no exceptionally bad pain or symptoms that would make her cry out. No bodily fluids were streaming down her legs or soiling her clothing, good because she was not bleeding, not out of control of her bodily functions, nor breaking her water right there before me. Her belly looked like the pregnancy was about 20 to 25 weeks along, good *and* bad because most problems for women not in extreme pain in that early stage of pregnancy were usually minor: urinary tract infections, stomach bugs, ligament pain, a musculoskeletal injury. If something was wrong or emergent, like unstoppable preterm labor, serious infection, or rupture of membranes, the baby was almost certainly non-viable. Things could get pretty bad pretty quickly.

All that was going through my head just as she arrived at the door. I went over to assess and interview her, do my exam, and formulate a plan based on my findings. Ms. Z told me she was 23 years old and that this was her first pregnancy. She had had regular prenatal care in our hospital clinic without complications. The previous day she had started to feel low level abdominal pain that came and went but never got too bad. When the pain didn't go away as she was trying to go to sleep, she thought she should come in. That's it. The whole history.

Now my work was to get the real story, to ask all the pertinent positives and negatives that would help me decide how much of an exam to do, how quickly to do it, and what our next steps should be. To my questions, her replies were: no fever, no nausea, no vomiting, no pain with urination, no bleeding, no discharge, no recent sexual activity, no headache, no recent trauma, no change in pain with rest or with activity, and some recognition of baby's movement, but not much. Her responses did not help identify the source of the pain.

The next step was the exam and checking the well-being of the baby. I measured Ms. Z's abdomen, which was the appropriate size for a 22-week pregnancy, and listened to the baby's heartbeat with a Doppler. It was fine, steady at 150 beats per minute. I did the always-necessary pelvic exam. Upper-level residents say if a woman presents to Labor and Delivery with a complaint, she never leaves without a pelvic exam. "Even for a sore throat?" I had asked, horrified! Yes, the worst thing that might happen in triaging her would be a pelvic problem, or bleeding, or labor, or an infection that would affect the pregnancy would be missed because the pelvic exam had been omitted.

A pelvic exam was necessary for Ms. Z's case since the cause of her discomfort was still unclear from taking the history. I did the pelvic. I will never forget what that felt like. The pelvic exam is done to check a patient's cervix. Many reasons require this check: to see if the cervix is tender, which would signal infection, or open, which would signal preterm labor or an incompetent cervix, or to see if there is blood, or discharge, or amniotic fluid present, all things that would help answer questions about the cause of the patient's symptoms. This time when I examined, I did not know exactly what I was feeling. When I was gently trying to assess the cervix, I was met immediately by what felt like a huge smooth water-balloon-like structure, that was filling the entire vagina. While my fingers were still trying to locate what felt like a cervix, I felt something that startled me, because it was actually moving — definite little jolting, worm-like movements that were separate from anything Ms. Z was doing.

My neutral doctor face probably dissolved because I had never felt anything like this. I immediately called my second-year resident to come down to the triage area for something emergent, and she did. When she did her own exam, she confirmed what I probably already knew — this was the bulging amniotic sac — coming through a mostly-open cervix — with tiny little legs in the sac, bending and stretching, kicking around, unaware anything was going on that shouldn't be. This was an emergency. Just because the patient didn't look or sound emergent didn't mean her situation wasn't a true emergency.

The second year resident quickly explained the situation to Ms. Z, with the important decisions she would have to quickly make concerning the future of her pregnancy.

If we did nothing, Ms. Z would most certainly lose the pregnancy. A 22 week pregnancy is not viable, and would not be viable for at least a few more weeks. In the early 1990s when this happened, 25 weeks was considered the very beginning of viability. That would be with the best medical and neonatal intensive care services available. Her cervix was already about 5 centimeters open, and the amniotic sac with parts of the baby were poking through the cervix, creating an hourglass.

If we did nothing, the sac would soon likely spontaneously rupture, and the cervix would open on its own, expelling a non-viable baby. If the patient wanted everything done to try to save her baby, we could offer to place her in a steep Trendelenburg position, with her feet elevated and head down. The position would allow gravity to attempt to help the amniotic sac recede through the cervix. We would be giving her medication to relax the uterus. We would then take her to the OR to place a cerclage, which is a purse-string suture through the cervix, to attempt to keep the cervix closed for the rest of the pregnancy, or at least long enough to create a viable pregnancy.

We explained this intervention was no guarantee of success. The head-down position may not work, or the medication may not work. The procedure itself could cause a problem, like rupturing the amniotic sac or tearing the cervix, causing bleeding or infection. Even if the procedure was initially successful, the baby would not be viable for weeks. The pregnancy could end at any time before viability, or at the cusp of viability. The baby could be born with numerous medical problems from prematurity.

Ms. Z needed to decide quickly as time was of the essence. Her significant other came into the room for a detailed discussion with the upper-level residents and the attending who was on call that night. After a lengthy and detailed discussion, Ms. Z decided on choice number two: to have everything done to save her baby. We went into action.

Since the night time shift was almost almost over, the procedure would be planned for the first thing in the morning. Much preparation was needed: IV fluids and antibiotics to get running; bloodwork to do as when anyone would be going to the OR; an official ultrasound to measure just how big the baby was; how much fluid was actually there and where it was; checking the placental location; assessing if the baby appeared healthy and did not have some major abnormality, which could alter Ms. Z's decision to try to do everything, or that might affect the possible outcome; medications to be given to relax the uterus, to give gravity some time to work to move that amniotic sac back into the uterus where it belonged. Once all that was done, the patient was ready to be taken to the OR.

I was a first year resident. Ms. Z could not be considered my case. She was the domain of the most experienced resident, who was to be guided by the attending physician. The night-time fourth year resident was going to stay to perform the procedure. I was the one who had first admitted Ms. Z, so I was invited to stay and participate in whatever minimal way they needed me. I felt Ms. Z *was* my patient. To leave just as she was about to go into the OR for a scary procedure after I had been with her throughout the night, explaining, discussing, examining, and making preparations would seem like a dump to the next resident coming on-shift and a break in her continuity of care.

I stayed. This wasn't the first or the last time I would stay on past my shift for something interesting or from the obligation I felt to see this through. We took Ms. Z to the OR. The anesthesiologist gave her a spinal anesthetic so she would be numb from the waist down. She was also given enough sedating medicine to lessen her anxiety, so she was not acutely aware of everything going on during the procedure. She was prepped and cleaned, and we were finally ready to take another look to see what was even possible. I technically did little more than hold a retractor and hand instruments to the more experienced resident, but we saw that the sac had almost completely receded back up past the cervix. Now we were looking at something that looked a bit like a donut, with a hole in the middle. This was a hole that should not have been there. Looking right up into that hole we could still see the bottom part of the amniotic sac. By putting gentle clamps on the cervical edges, the resident was able to ever-so-carefully place the two purse-string sutures made of a permanent material, in-and-out, at various locations around the edges of the cervix, and in the end, tie them in a knot so they would keep the cervix closed if everything went as planned.

Watching was fascinating. There was minimal bleeding, no ruptured amniotic membranes, and seemingly, no complications. The plan was to keep Ms. Z in the hospital on bedrest until the team felt there was no infection, no bleeding, and no contractions, and that she would be able to go home on a similar regimen of greatly restricted activity. We were not sure how long that would be, but the first 48 hours would be critical.

I went home about noon, exhausted but hopeful. Although no one said this was my case, **I** was still the one to write all the orders, do the dictation, sign the patient out to the first year resident that was already on-shift, and make sure the plan was clear to everyone before I could leave.

Two nights later, I was doing paperwork on a relatively quiet night shift when I got a call from the antepartum floor, where all the pregnant patients who needed to be hospitalized were stationed. Patients had various medical problems: high blood pressure that needed monitoring, infections, and preterm labor. This was where Ms. Z had been placed following her procedure. She had been stable since the morning of the surgery and was being closely monitored on strict bedrest. When I was paged and saw the extension of the antepartum unit in my beeper, my heart skipped a beat. "You better come here right away!" the nurse said. Never a good request to hear.

Ms. Z was asleep and was suddenly awakened by a sensation of something wet under her in the bed. She called the nurse, who pulled back the sheets and was shocked to see a moderate amount of blood mixed with what must have been a large amount of greenish amniotic fluid. I ran over to the unit. In my calmest way possible I gently looked under the sheets. I told Ms. Z that this was not good, and we needed to get her somewhere other than her dimly lit hospital room, to take a thorough look at what had happened. I called my more senior residents, and both of them came to the OR to meet us as I was wheeling her in. Ms. Z was softly crying on her rolling hospital bed. We had the anesthesiologist stand-by in case we needed him. When we got the patient into the proper position to do an exam, there was no mistaking what we saw: blood, clots, and a green thick fluid called meconium, which is a sign of distress, that is released into the amniotic sac when a baby is fighting to stay alive.

What we saw, what told us that this was the end for this patient and this baby, was unmistakable. We saw two tiny, perfect, beautiful baby feet, like doll's feet, lying still, peeking out of the vagina. I started to cry. I couldn't help myself. From the beginning I knew the odds were poor for saving this pregnancy. I knew this could be the outcome. A baby this small, this premature, was unlikely to make it through all the weeks and months of challenges after such a difficult start. It all just hit me when I saw the two tiny feet.

We had tried our best and had honored her request to have everything done, but everything was not enough. This was not the first time I had seen a patient or her baby meet a bad outcome, but it was the first time I had been intimately involved in every step through the life-and-then-the-death process. On further inspection and with adequate anesthesia assistance, we could see the cerclage did tear through her cervix. This was causing bleeding from the areas where the stitch caused too much strain on the tissue, which was determined to stretch and open.

Connected to those two tiny perfect feet, was the tiny perfect body of a tiny perfect 22 week old fetus — with arms and legs and fused eyelids and mostly transparent skin, lying silently, as if asleep, practically falling out of the open cervix once we cut the knots in the straining sutures. The tiny, flat, bloodless umbilical cord was still attached to the placenta, which, luckily, completely and spontaneously expelled from the uterus as well. We detached the placenta, and placed the bruised but intact baby in a tiny open plastic box, with a little hat and blanket, since it was possible Ms. Z would want to see her baby when we were finished.

We repaired the torn cervix, making sure there was no active bleeding and no placental parts left in the uterus. We gave Ms. Z the appropriate antibiotics to prevent infection and medications so the uterus would remain contracted to lessen her bleeding. We called the clergy she had requested, and cleaned her up so she could go back to her room to spend some time with her family and make the arrangements.

I needed to talk with Ms. Z. I tried to remember that part of my care would be to talk to her about exactly what happened and that it was nothing she had done or didn't do. We had to discuss what her risks would be for it to happen again with a future pregnancy, to explain that next time she would need to have a cerclage placed early in pregnancy, and about other types of monitoring and treatments she might need. I knew she might need a therapist to help with the grieving process, or she might need additional time to just talk to me or anyone else involved in her care.

That would come later. I needed to start by being there at her side, and expressing how truly sorry I was this had happened and acknowledging how it would take time to process all of this. Then, a few minutes later, my beeper went off. "The delivery room needs you. Someone is about to deliver."

6

Circumcisions — A Little Off the Top

The first half of my first year of residency I spent 13 weeks in the delivery room and 13 weeks doing a family planning rotation. Now I was heading into night rotation, where I was to go in to work every evening at 11, work through the night, and usually stay until the next day's morning clinic was over. This was the rotation with the most potential to screw up my body clock and my circadian rhythms. Somehow, though, I wasn't worried and was actually looking forward to it, since I knew I would be home (almost) every night to have dinner with my family and to put my kids to bed. Sometimes I thought having had two babies prepared me for residency, since they both involved getting very little sleep, and forever feeling like nothing I did was ever good enough.

The fourth year night resident met me in the delivery room the first night of our rotation, where we took sign-out from the daytime team. After going over all the information on the currently laboring patients, and writing our notes, she told me to meet her in the nursery, where all the newborn babies were.

The new policy was all of the boy babies who were supposed to be circumcised would be done by the night shift. The responsibility of the first year night time resident on rotation was to perform all the circumcisions. Since this was a new policy, I hadn't yet learned how to do a circumcision. My fourth year resident, Dr. S, was pretty matter-of-fact about it, and determined to show me how to do it. Her approach was see-one-do-one-teach-one, as was the case for so many things I had so far learned. The number of babies to be circumcised, or circ'ed as we came to call them, varied from one to six each night, depending on how many boy babies were born and how many families wanted circumcisions. It was not for me to comment, or discuss, or even speak to the parents about circumcision. Consents had been signed during the day, and were the responsibility of the daytime first year Labor and Delivery room resident to explain and obtain. We just had to make sure there was a signed and witnessed consent on the baby's chart before actually performing the procedure.

I met Dr. S in the nursery, which looked like a small baby-assembly line. Four babies in cribs were lined up, waiting their turn. When we were ready to start, the nurse picked up the first baby, identified him by his name bands, and looked for the consent form his mother had signed. All was in place. She next positioned the baby on the appropriately-named circumcision-board, where his arms and legs were restrained. Dr. S explained, "So he doesn't kick us when we have a scalpel in our hands." Note to self: we do not want to be kicked by a baby when we are about to use a sharp instrument on his delicate boy parts.

My resident-teacher laid out all her instruments, and methodically and in sterile fashion, went through all the many steps of a circumcision, explaining how she does what she does. The procedure was interesting, and in the end, successful, but the baby was screaming the entire time. I couldn't understand why they did not use any anesthetic when doing a procedure that was so obviously painful for the baby.

Dr. S told me that the baby was already so uncomfortable from being restrained on the board, so as long as the procedure was done quickly, there was not much additional discomfort for the baby. I didn't think that was true. I watched her methodically perform the rest of the circumcisions that evening, trying to keep the steps in order in my head. I was sure the next night would be my turn. Every time a baby was touched by or with something that would seem to cause pain, the baby did scream louder and longer. How could Dr. S and the nurses not see that? I wondered if there was anything they could do since I was uncomfortable with the idea of doing something to a baby that was screaming in pain. Guess I wouldn't have made a good pediatrician, since that is a lot of what they do.

I wasn't sure I'd be able to do a circumcision properly if I was always thinking about doing it faster to limit the baby's discomfort. The next day I called the hospital pharmacy to see if there was anything I could order to make the procedure less painful for the baby. Yes, the pharmacy had an anesthetic cream we could apply to the penis about a half hour prior to the circumcision for numbing.

I told my fourth year resident, and she said, "OK, but you're going to have to go over there and apply it yourself." This was her way of telling me the nurses in the nursery were so busy that the last thing they wanted was more work, especially something they had to do on multiple babies. They would have to keep the timing in mind so that the anesthetic cream would be applied to all the babies at exactly the right time, a half hour before their turn on the board. I decided to try the cream, partly because I thought the anesthesia would make my job easier, and partly because I had a son. I would have wanted someone to do that for him in a similar circumstance. In reality, my son had had a *bris*, which is the Jewish version of the circumcision, done on the eighth day of a baby boy's life, at home, during which the baby is actually given some wine during the procedure, which is our anesthetic equivalent. Just for the record, I didn't watch my son's circumcision.

After thinking about how I could get the anesthetic cream on the babies in the right time interval, and in an effective, efficient manner, I came up with what I thought was a brilliant idea. I decided to carry it out starting the very next night. I came in for the night rotation about 20 minutes early, and looked at the list of babies awaiting circumcision that night. I put my plan into action, with some minor assistance from the nursery nurses, whom, it turned out, were all in favor of making babies less uncomfortable during their procedures.

We kept the cream a secret. When I returned later that night with my fourth year resident, imagine her surprise when, in removing the first baby's diaper, she found a pacifier, full of anesthetic cream, parked strategically over the baby's penis, allowing the medicine to take effect. The hospital had special pacifiers for newborns, which were shaped in such a way that when placed in a baby's mouth, a finger could be placed in the hole, to hold it in place. It was in this hole I had placed the anesthetic cream, and then put the pacifier in place over the penis, held in place by the diaper. Brilliant! Numbing and protection in one!

The cream in the pacifier could stay there between 30 to 60 minutes, so that when we came to do the procedure, there had been time for the anesthetic to take effect. Maybe it was my imagination, but starting that night, the babies cried less during the circumcisions. Note to self: try to always get there on time to place the pacifiers as this would become yet another job for first year residents — yay!

7

I Can Help You Remove That

In the second week of my gynecology rotation, a patient was waiting for an exam in a clinic cubicle. When I first saw Ms. L I thought she must be in the wrong clinic. She was young, mid-thirties, and lying on the exam table she looked as if she was 9 months pregnant. Her belly jutted out as far as a full term baby. I started my history-taking and exam, but was not sure how to approach the large belly that was obviously the reason she was there in the first place. Turns out, it was the reason; and my work-up began.

I asked Ms. L the standard questions and wrote her information down. She was 36, single, from Mexico, and spoke some English. She had no children and no complaints other than her belly feeling big: no pain, no fevers, no medical issues, and heavy regular periods. She felt full very fast when she ate. I had learned enough to do a systematic review from head-to-toe when I did my exam: head, eyes, ears, neck, lungs, heart, and abdomen, which was huge, firm, protruding and not necessarily tender. Ms. L's abdomen was obviously not normal. I wasn't sure if she was aware of this mass that was filling her abdominal cavity. She seemed like it was just "there." It didn't seem to cause her pain, but definite discomfort.

When I did my pelvic exam, I found a large, immobile, centrally located enlarged structure in the middle of her pelvis; I was not yet skilled enough to know what I was feeling exactly, but I did what I always did, and presented her to my more senior resident. I told him that it seemed like this may be a surgical case. His eyes got wide, and he said, "Well, let's go see." He was impressed with the size of the mass, and how nonplussed Ms. L seemed. Once we decided that this was a potential surgical case, we had to decide, that is, *I* had to decide, what the proper differential diagnosis would be, and what the proper work up would consist of to get her to the OR. Ms. L needed lab work, scans, and a discussion of the types of surgery available to her and why. The proper people had to be assembled. We had to be sure Ms. L was healthy enough to undergo surgery, and we had to be aware of the various things we might find.

The differential diagnosis of a large pelvic mass: The mass could be ovarian or uterine cancer, or a benign, non cancerous tumor on either the ovaries or the uterus. Other possibilities included a large cyst, a mass in her intestines, a large abscess or infection, a pregnancy related condition, a cancer of the fallopian tubes or of the urinary bladder, a foreign body, enlarged lymph nodes, fibroids in the uterus, or several other more unusual things. My job was to do enough tests so when we finally did take her to the OR we were fairly sure what we were going to find, who we needed there to help us, and what would happen to her afterward. I made my list and my presentation, set about ordering everything we needed, and explained all this to the patient in the best way I knew how.

After the work-up and discussion, Ms. L's surgery day finally came. This was a case for the most senior resident, with an attending physician, and me as the second assistant, along with a medical student who was rotating through. I was the first year resident with the major responsibility for getting the patient ready for the operation, presenting her to the fourth year resident, and assisting in the OR with whatever anyone needed. I was also supposed to be teaching the medical student along the way.

I was luckily in a position to delegate some of the scut to the student, which I happily did, but I was still responsible for everything he did. Ms. L's lab work was done. The tumor markers were negative. We were probably not going to find cancer, although that was still possible. A pelvic sonogram showed the large mass we were feeling was most likely a very enlarged uterus, seemingly the size of a 6 month pregnancy, only without a baby inside. The CAT scan showed the mass likely did not involve other organs, like her liver, intestines, or kidneys.

Ms. L seemed healthy enough to undergo a major surgery. She had signed her consent to remove the mass, possibly her uterus, possibly one or both ovaries, and any other procedure deemed necessary. That is how patients signed their consents back then, explaining that in case we found something unexpected in there once the surgery started, we had their permission to do whatever we needed. In the present day, we rarely would be able to have someone agree to just leave it all up to us.

We assembled in the OR. I held Ms. L's hand as she fell asleep from the anesthesia. I was the one who had the most contact with her, and it just felt right that I should be the last person she would see before going under general anesthesia. Note to self: in the OR, hold her hand and be the last person my surgical patient sees before she falls asleep.

Once Ms. L was asleep and uncovered, we could see that from her small frame, this huge round mass protruded even more than before, making it appear as if she had somehow swallowed a basketball. The fourth year resident and the attending went about discussing what type of incision they would need to make, and what their technique would be like, depending on what they found inside. I was listening but not involved in the decision making. They asked me several questions to see if I had prepared for the surgery. What layers would we be cutting through? What blood vessels supply the various layers? What instruments would we be using? Luckily I knew most of the answers. If I hadn't they would be likely to tell me to just leave the OR since that would have signaled I really wasn't ready. Once the patient was prepped and draped, we were ready to begin.

Standing at the OR table was the team. In the primary surgeon spot was the fourth year resident, Dr. P, a tall, broad-shouldered man, about 32. I knew him quite well by then. He was a kind of love-him-or-hate-him guy, rough around the edges, as my father used to say. Dr. P liked to joke around, sometimes inappropriately, but was a good doctor and a good surgeon. Then there was Dr. F, the second year resident across the table from Dr. P, the first assistant as she was called. She was younger and petite — a no-nonsense person, who was one year ahead of me. We were friendly, but I was acutely aware of the fact that my role remained as a subordinate to her, whether I knew as much as she did or not. She too had this awareness. The attending physician stood off to the side, watching everything that was going on, but not feeling obligated to scrub in or put on gloves unless something unplanned occurred. Then there was me next to the first assistant. I was scrubbed in, designated as the second assistant. Actually this is the equivalent of the retractor holder, the suture cutter, and, if I was lucky, the closer.

Once all the difficult parts of the operation were done, the primary surgeon and the first assistant sometimes let the second assistant have the privilege of placing some of the closing sutures in the layers of fascia, peritoneum, fat, and subcutaneous tissue that all were closed individually back then. Whether or not the second assistant got to do any of that was completely dependent on the primary and the first assistant: how much they trusted you, how much they felt like taking the extra time to teach you how to do the work, and even, what mood they were in at that moment.

Dr. P made a vertical incision in the skin, from right under the patient's belly button to the top of her pubic bone. From there, the two surgeons worked together in a series of planned, well-orchestrated moves, to dissect down through the tissues and the fascia, using a combination of a scalpel, electricity, and other sharp instruments. Along the way they stopped to give me directions, or orders, or to ask me questions about the different structures we were seeing and the blood vessels, nerves, and muscles in the pelvis. Once the fascia and the peritoneum were opened, we saw a huge structure jutting out in the midline. This was her uterus, about the size of a 6-month pregnancy.

I was shocked. I had never seen a uterus this big that didn't have a baby inside. I was amazed at how easily they were able to pop the whole thing out anteriorly, through the incision, as the top portion was seemingly not attached to very much inside. We could trace her fallopian tubes to the ovaries and locate the various ligaments that were surrounding this huge uterus. They pointed them out to me while at the same time asking me what I would do here, or there, and how I would proceed in a case such as this. I had studied, so I usually knew the answers, thank goodness. They slowly and methodically interrupted all the blood supply to the uterus, the surgeons working on the structures on their own side, being assisted by the surgeon across the table.

After about 25 minutes, the entire structure was removed, leaving a big space where it had been. I had seen a few hysterectomies before. I tried not to let on how excited and how amazed I still was to watch something like this going on and to participate in the process. After it was ascertained that there was no active bleeding, they began the closure. Dr. P said to Dr. F, "Switch places," meaning she and I should rearrange ourselves at the table so I was now directly across from him, which we did. He proceeded to lead me through the entire closure procedure, allowing me to place all the sutures, commenting on how I should hold the needle-holder, and the other instruments. "Follow the curve of the needle," he would say. "Use your instrument to lift the tissue." "Use the tip of the clamp."

At last the final stitch was placed. The attending was long-gone by then, and the second year resident had scrubbed out to write the orders, which I would have had to do when we were done. Dr. F was good that way. I glanced over at the anesthesiologist during the closure. He was obviously annoyed that this was taking twice as long as usual because I was learning how to do it all, but I didn't care. Dr. P didn't seem to care either. We finished. I placed the bandage over the patient's belly with a true sense of accomplishment. I did not even realize how much my neck and back were aching from standing in that position for over two hours. Note to self: use a step-stool when all the other surgeons are taller than you!

8

Every 73 Seconds

On one of my last on-call nights as a first year resident, I was sitting at a computer in the lounge area, when my second year resident, Dr. R, came in. "We need to go down to the ER," she said, "A rape case came in." I immediately got up from my chair. In all the on-calls and all the nights in the hospital, I had never been the resident called to the ER for a rape case. Second year residents were generally called to the ER. I had gone with the second year resident when I had no first year duties to perform, which was almost never. This time the second year resident, realizing that this was my opportunity for learning what to do and how to manage a rape case, said she would accompany me. My responsibility was to assist and learn to do whatever was needed.

On our way to the ER, Dr. R, the second year resident said that when a woman came in to the ER after a reported rape, we were never sure what we were going to find. We were always expected to do the same things, to follow a very specific list of requirements, both medically and legally. In this case, we found a sad, quiet 25-year-old woman, wrapped in a blanket, crying softly and sitting on a gurney. Dr. R and I stopped for two minutes at the desk outside her curtain to get the brief story from the uniformed policewoman stationed there, and to pick up a rape kit.

The kit was a cardboard box that contained all the evidence-gathering materials we would need to collect and log everything in a specific way. Dr. R had been through this methodical procedure numerous times. She knew what to do without reading the instructions on the box. We went into the curtained room, and tried to gently and softly ask Ms. M what had happened. I was documenting everything she said, and could see she had already repeated this story several times. We listened.

Ms. M was out with her friends. Everyone was drinking. She did not feel she drank that much. A friend of a friend had offered her a ride home. The next thing she remembered was waking up somewhere outside, feeling bruised and missing some of her clothes. An ambulance was called and Ms. M was brought to the ER. Our job was to listen and collect evidence. The rest was a police matter. Dr. R was kind but official. She explained that to best create a case, we needed to collect as much evidence as we could. Although much of the process would be uncomfortable, we would try to work as quickly and thoroughly as possible.

Ms. M agreed, and we went to work. We had to break the seal on the rape kit. Each of the ten different collection envelopes in the kit had instructions on what to collect and how. Over the next fifteen minutes, we methodically collected swabs and samples and hairs and cultures and scrapings from various parts of her body. Dr. R would stop periodically and softly explain, "I need to remove a few hairs, and I know it will sting but I'll be quick" or "I'm going to gently run this brush over your skin now."

I understood how women could say that sometimes the collection feels like another assault, even when done by the most empathetic health care practitioners. Every potential area where there may be evidence or DNA from the attacker had to be swabbed and probed, placed in an evidence envelope in a certain way, and catalogued carefully so that the chain of evidence was not violated, and that eventually an actual case could be brought against someone, using these collections. Ms. M's clothing had to be collected and bagged. We gave her hospital scrubs to wear. She was offered testing and treatment for various infections and sexually transmitted diseases, including HIV, since there was no way of knowing what she had been exposed to. When we were done, a rape crisis counselor came to speak with Ms. M and offer follow up services. The whole episode was overwhelming and scary. I could not imagine how many times Dr. R would have had to go through this entire routine to be so automatic following the procedures. I also could not imagine a victim having to go through this with anyone with less empathy and kindness than Dr. R.

Once that entire procedure was done, Dr. R and I were able to talk. I asked how she stayed unemotional while performing all those horrible, invasive tasks, with the patient crying the entire time. She told me that she just keeps telling herself to do all the collection properly and make sure during the entire process to get all the evidence that would be needed to identify and prosecute the perpetrator. If she could do that, she knew she'd be doing the most to help this woman in the future. If she were unable to do her job, then somehow later she would be responsible for not having properly collected the necessary evidence. Dr. R wasn't unsympathetic; she just knew how she could do the most good. Note to self: always be thorough, empathetic, non judgemental and do the most good.

9

Of Course I Believe in Choice, but It's Not as Simple as That

Making rounds on the antepartum service, I would see all the pregnant patients needing to be managed in an in-the-hospital setting. One young woman I will never forget, Thalia. She has given me the okay to use her name. Thalia was almost 24 weeks pregnant with her first baby. Several days before she was admitted, she woke up in a pool of fluid. We determined that Thalia's water had broken, very prematurely. In the obstetrical world, we called this PPROM, the acronym for preterm, premature rupture of membranes. PPROM occurs when the amniotic sac ruptures very distant from the baby being fully grown and before the start of labor. Once PPROM is determined, there are many things we, as her providers must do — from counseling her about the potential, mostly poor, outcomes, to doing numerous tests to decide what those outcomes are most likely to be.

When Thalia was admitted, we had done cultures to check for infection since infection is the number one reason water may break early. We had done an ultrasound to see if there was indeed any fluid still left in the amniotic sac since sometimes, even when the water breaks, more fluid can reaccumulate. We had done numerous blood tests to see if there were signs of other complications. While we were waiting for the test results, we counseled her extensively about the possible outcomes when the amniotic sac ruptures too early.

Amniotic fluid has many positive effects on the growing fetus. When the placenta is functioning and healthy the amniotic fluid level is usually normal. Chemicals in the amniotic fluid help the baby's lungs to properly mature. Amniotic fluid provides a cushioning around the baby to allow room for growth and movement of the body and limbs. The fluid protects the baby from the world outside and prevents infection.

When the fluid is gone too early, so is the protection and the other growth and development benefits. Once the amniotic sac has ruptured, the most likely course of events is that within the next few days, labor will spontaneously begin in an attempt to empty the uterus, whatever the gestational age of the baby. All this provided a huge dilemma for Thalia and for the team caring for her. While initially most patients with preterm complications want everything done for their babies, this baby was only 23 plus weeks old, which at that time, was on the cusp of being viable. Even in the best-case scenario, with no other complications, a 23 week old baby would be looking at a lot of problems on the outside. This was something we had to think about carefully. We decided to wait for all the test results before making any decisions.

Thalia remained in the hospital for a few days, mostly on bedrest. We monitored her vital signs and temperature, checking for signs of infection and waiting for the test results. When the results came back, we had to have one of the toughest discussions with her that I have ever been a party to. Her blood tests started to show an increasing white blood count, which was a sign of infection. The most likely place for an infection to occur was inside the uterus since the amniotic sac was already broken. The infectious cultures, which were taken directly from the amniotic fluid, would show us exactly the type of infection. Two of the cultures were positive, meaning infections were present. One was gonorrhea; one was herpes. These two sexually transmitted diseases must have been transmitted from a partner, who got them from someone else.

The horrific news, in addition to the obvious information that her partner had other partners, was that either or both infections were likely to cause severe developmental problems in the baby, especially at this premature stage. There could and likely would be brain damage, developmental problems, possible blindness, and lung, liver, and skin problems. Other problems would come from the extreme prematurity of the baby if it were to be born soon: poor lung development, possible deafness, poor motor function, and other disabilities. Thalia was likely looking at a poor outcome no matter what happened. She was currently at a gestational age considered on the cusp of viability, even in ideal circumstances. When she entered the hospital, the idea was to do everything to keep her baby inside, gestating, and growing, until it was old enough to live in the outside world with some assistance.

Now that her water was broken, although Thalia had not yet gone into labor, and with the known infections and the likely outcome for the baby, the best option was probably to get the baby out of there before the infections affected Thalia's well-being. In all of this, one of the biggest dilemmas, was that if we all agreed and decided that for Thalia's benefit, the baby should be delivered, what would we do if the baby came out compromised but alive, with a heartbeat?

At 24 weeks, the hospital would be obligated to resuscitate the baby and place it on a respirator, regardless of the serious medical issues the baby would likely have. If another patient had come into the hospital in a similar situation but without these known infections, and I had seen a few by now, then of course we would do all we could to assist the baby in its transition to the outside world: warming, ventilating, feeding through a tube, giving medication. We would do anything the parents wanted done to help an extremely premature baby live and thrive. In this case, where the baby, already compromised, and highly likely to suffer many long term, life-long disabilities, the thought was a little different. We always asked ourselves if doing all that we could was the right thing to do, and we asked that here as well. Present at the counseling session that we had with Thalia were the high-risk obstetrician, several pediatricians, including specialists in premature babies, neonatologists, a specialist in infectious diseases, and a perinatal counselor.

To make matters worse, Thalia told us that her partner was no longer in the picture. He had left her several weeks prior to her admission. She might not be in a financial or emotional state to take on the life long responsibilities of a severely compromised baby. We had to offer her options, which we did.

The first option was to continue to wait, hoping labor would spontaneously begin. She was seemingly already moving toward infection. The baby was living in a place that had cultured positive for some pretty bad current infections, in spite of treatment. Thalia may soon labor on her own and deliver the baby. However, she was also beginning to have a rising white blood cell count, some tenderness in her abdomen, and a slightly fast heart rate, tachycardia. Waiting was not the best option since Thalia could then end up septic, and very sick or dead. We advised against this option.

The second option was to induce her to deliver, as usually a premature uterus already infected will be sensitive to our augmentation medications. Thalia would likely go into labor and deliver the baby in a short time. Getting the baby out was of course indicated. The sooner the baby was removed from her uterus, the better chance Thalia would have to avoid major infectious consequences. The problem with this choice was that once the induction of labor was underway, the baby would likely not tolerate her labor contractions, being as premature and as compromised as it already was. What if we see, on a fetal monitor, that the baby was crashing, as we call it in Labor and Delivery? Do we intervene and do a C section on a baby that was highly unlikely to survive, let alone to survive with any real quality of life? Do we do a C section on an infected uterus that will more likely result in worse infection for the mother? Now that we would have introduced surgery on a uterus unlikely to respond well to surgery, there would be so much bleeding, and maybe enough that she would end up with a transfusion, or worse, a hysterectomy? Then Thalia's chance for future pregnancy would be gone. Along with the other possible outcome from this choice, if we induced her, and somehow the baby tolerated the labor, and was born vaginally, with any heartbeat at all, it would be resuscitated by hospital protocol. Resuscitation on an infected micro-preemie would likely be painful, ineffective, and excruciating for all. And if the baby survived the efforts, then what? Likely a long, drawn-out NICU stay with poor chance of survival, and many future procedures and long term problems.

A third option to present, but an option knowing all of the other possible outcomes, was offered to Thalia: to consider the procedure as a termination of pregnancy. There was a way to make sure that the baby did not come out alive and with a heart beat. Then the resuscitation part would not be necessary. The monitoring would not be necessary. Thoughts about other interventions would not be necessary. If the baby were no longer alive inside her, then the procedure to remove the baby would be done with the patient fully sedated and mostly unaware.

Thalia would not have to fully experience labor and would not have to feel movements or be on a monitor in the process. This would essentially be a termination of her pregnancy; a removal of an infected nidus, an area of focus where bacteria have multiplied, causing an infection. Then we would continue to treat her for a very bad infection, until she was, hopefully, well again.

I listened, as the attendings discussed how this could be done. Until this meeting, I hadn't known about option three. They explained that they could use a medication that would essentially stop the baby's heart while it was still inside her. Then her labor would be immediately induced until the now not-alive baby would be removed in a procedure that might be carried out with or without instruments to be sure the baby and the entire placenta, which were all involved in the intra-uterine infection, would be totally removed.

Thalia listened intently, as the two attendings told her about this option. They explained that she could be totally sedated and comfortable throughout, and as aware or un-aware as she wanted; that she would be in a room distant from where women were laboring and having their "normal" labors and deliveries, with all their attendant happy noises and celebrations. No one was unaware that what they were asking, what they were recommending, was that she actively participate in ending her baby's life, to save her own, and to avoid the other probable outcomes that they had described to her. As this realization swept over her, she began to cry. Just listening to the discussion, I almost did as well. She asked if she could think and talk to her family. Of course she could.

All I could think about while we were waiting for her response was how incredibly difficult this decision must be. I thought about the continuing debate and controversy on the subject of abortion and all the political protesters, both for and against abortion. I wondered how many of those protesters have ever found themselves in this situation. Not many I would guess. I was again certain that no one except a woman and her doctor should be able to decide. No one can decide what is right for someone else in this situation. This would be a decision that would be agonized over, mulled over, cried over, and played and replayed in Thalia's head and heart probably for the rest of her life. She had all the information on all the possibilities. Time was running out for her safety.

After thinking about the possible outcomes, Thalia decided to terminate her pregnancy. We explained how this would be done, and the high risk Ob specialist and I went into her room the next morning. The procedure required the instillation of potassium chloride (KCl) in an injectable syringe that would be inserted through her abdomen with a long needle under ultrasound guidance. The goal was to find the baby's heart and instill the KCl. This would stop the heart from beating. The baby would no longer be alive.

Thalia was sad, but resolved. She had been considering what was about to happen ever since she had been given the information about the possible outcomes. We once again explained the procedure, and had her sign consent forms. Dr. W, the high-risk Ob doctor, swabbed her exposed belly with Betadine. My job was to place the sonogram machine on her abdomen to look for the heart. Looking at this screen I couldn't help but think about how, usually, all anyone wants to see when a sonogram is done is that small flash of light, the proof that a living being with a heartbeat is in there.

Usually everything changes in that minute you see the heartbeat. Here we weren't looking for the heart beat to confirm a pregnancy, or as a cause for celebration. We needed to see that heart beat so we knew where to stick the needle. Once we instilled the KCl, we would watch that heart beat, watch it slow down until the blinking light was no more. I stared at the screen. I turned it away from Thalia so she didn't see or hear what was going on in real time, although she was aware. I watched the blink-blink-blink of the heart beat, and, as professional as I tried to be, when I saw that heartbeat cease, the hair stood up on the back of my neck. I had to turn away from the screen.

I knew this was the best choice under the circumstances. I knew that this was the lesser of evils. I knew that we were doing this mother and this infant a service and giving Thalia a choice to avoid potential sepsis and delivery of a severely compromised very premature baby. I knew all this. Yet I couldn't help but tear up when the light went out. How could I not? I thought of all the babies I had delivered. I thought of my own babies. I thought of babies everywhere. My specialty is The Happy Specialty, except when it's not.

Once that distasteful part of this multi-part procedure was done, the next part was fairly standard. I had already done it many times during the course of my residency. When a baby is not alive inside the uterus and is over 20 weeks in gestation, the delivery must proceed like any other delivery. Medications meant to induce labor — strong, regular uterine contractions, were given until the contractions were frequent and strong enough to dilate the cervix, and the baby could be delivered. In this case, however, there would be no monitoring, no pediatrician needed, and no jubilant ending. The patient was given strong sedating and strong pain medications so she could go through her labor mostly unaware. She also needed other medications to counteract the side effects of the induction medications, the nausea, vomiting, diarrhea, and fever, and more antibiotics for the now-established infection.

Thalia wanted family members with her as she drifted in and out of wakefulness. Various medical people came and went as well: nurses, counselors, residents, and the high-risk attending doctor. All played a part in her management. After about 16 hours, even through all of her pain and sedating meds, we could tell that the delivery was imminent. We had warned her that she may still feel pressure to push, and would likely still have to do some of the work of the actual delivery. When the time came, she did. It didn't take much pushing to deliver such a small baby. When it emerged, I looked at the small, lifeless body that just lay there, still, as I performed all my usual maneuvers to detach the baby from the placenta as gently as I could.

"Be professional," I told myself. The baby had the distinct odor of infection, as did the placenta, reassuring me that we had done the right thing. I handed the baby off to the nurses, who had already discussed with Thalia whether she wanted to see or hold the baby. Luckily the entire placenta came out at once, which is not always the case in this situation. If it hadn't all come out I'd have had to try to get it out with instruments, something quite risky in a preterm, infected uterus. As if a sign that Thalia had been through enough, there was no need for instruments, and there wasn't much bleeding. We had just the formalities of examining the baby, and the placenta, treating the patient's infection and discomfort, and helping her to heal, both physically and emotionally, which would take time. Thalia decided she did want to see the baby, but not hold it. We wrapped it up in a small blanket, took some pictures in case she wanted them for a keepsake, and showed her the tiny lifeless baby in a small makeshift crib. She asked for medication to help her sleep. Of course we complied.

I was drained. We all were. The debriefing, a meeting for all the health care providers involved in Thalia's care, was later that day. Whenever an emotionally difficult event happened in our unit, we had an official meeting to discuss the treatment and outcome and how we had been affected. These meetings were important because we tended to get so busy taking care of patients that we often forgot to take care of ourselves, and to discuss the toll that these situations had on us, as healthcare providers and as human beings.

10

Surprise!

On one of my last nights on call as a third-year resident, I was witness to one of the most shocking events of my entire residency. At about 10 that night, I was sitting at the desk in the delivery room, taking inventory of the patients in labor, assessing which ones would deliver before we signed out to the night crew at 11. A few patients were in early labor, one becoming active, and one who was being monitored for her high blood pressure and not in labor at all. I thought we would be able to turn all of these patients over to the incoming night residents, without too much activity going on in the last hour. Then the red phone rang at the desk. This was the special phone the emergency room used to call us when they had a particularly emergent patient they were going to be wheeling up to the delivery room in a hurry, usually because the patient had showed up in the ER in dire circumstances or about to deliver.

The ER docs would rather that she did so on the third floor, with us, instead of down there on the first floor with them. I happened to be the closest resident to the phone.

The rule was the closest resident was to answer the red phone when it rang, so we all could quickly get ready for whatever they were sending our way. I picked it up, said, "Yeah, Dr. Levy. What have you got?"

The ER physician told me a tale I had heard a few times before. A young woman presented to the ER with acute abdominal pains and vomiting. She was a large woman, over 250 pounds, and spoke only Spanish. The ER has translators who had asked her many questions, very specifically if she was pregnant. She vehemently denied being pregnant. As her pain got worse and, since they did a pregnancy test, which was positive, and since she acted like a patient in labor, they called us, and decided to send her our way. Ms. T was being wheeled up to Labor and Delivery, on a gurney in the express elevator, landing right in the triage area. She was huffing and puffing like hundreds of other patients I had seen, but we had no information about her. We had no idea exactly how pregnant she was, or what type of medical conditions or problems she had. Ms. T obviously did not have any prenatal care since she was swearing there was no way she was pregnant. As I was hanging up the phone, the noise from the triage area got louder. We knew a delivery was imminent.

Right there on the gurney we normally used for evaluating the triage patients, her baby, all seven plus pounds of him, was born within minutes. The first year resident, who was used to emergency deliveries, fairly easily did the delivery, clamped and cut the umbilical cord. The baby was whisked away to be evaluated by the pediatricians. Ms. T stopped screaming. The flurry of activity taking place all around us died down. We decided to take the patient back to the delivery room to await the placenta and repair any damage done by the quick and unexpected birth. There didn't seem to be much blood. We took a collective deep breath, and started to ask, in our combined, best Spanish, all the usual questions we had not yet had the chance to ask.

Ms. T. told us she had irregular periods. Over the past four or five months she had seen a few periods, not really sure of the dates. She said she always weighed between 230 and 250 pounds, and hadn't noticed much weight gain specifically in the past several months. She denied being aware of fetal movement, contractions, or water breaking. She had two other children, ten and seven years old, and no known medical problems although she hadn't visited a doctor on any regular basis.

In the middle of this conversation while we were still getting her prepped to undergo removal of her placenta, which had not yet presented itself, and repair her small tears, the patient started breathing heavily, stronger, and faster. Ms. T was acting like she was once again having increasingly painful abdominal contractions. We thought this breathing was unusual, but sometimes when the placenta is ready to deliver, contractions get strong again for it to be expelled. This much pain was uncommon.

My first year resident, who was mainly responsible for this delivery and was sitting on the stool at the foot of the table suddenly yelled to me, "Oh my God, come over here right now!" I went running, as I was over in the non-sterile area of the room, doing the paperwork, and asking all the questions. When I got to the edge of the delivery table, and looked from his point of view, what went through my mind, and what came out of my mouth, was, "Holy shit."

Here were two feet and two legs, a second baby was about a quarter of the way out of this woman's vagina. I called for the fourth year resident, who had not been previously involved. I called for nurses and attendings and pediatricians and anyone else who could possibly come in to assist. Ms. T was obviously and uncontrollably trying to push this baby out. When I slightly regained my composure, I sat down on the stool, and repeatedly ran through in my mind everything I had been taught about delivery of a feet-first baby vaginally. I had done several, always a second twin, which this one obviously was. Although it would be ideal to do it in a calmer, more planned set of circumstances, time to stop and think was not an option.

The first baby had hopefully paved the way. I hoped this baby was smaller. I quickly gowned and gloved, wrapped a towel around the lower half of the baby, which was out to about the waist, legs kicking. I gently held the lower half in one hand, and reached up to sweep one arm down. I turned the baby so I could do the same with the other arm, and then lifted the baby in the air by its legs, flexed the chin, and directed the patient to push as hard as she could and pop! Out popped the baby's head. She looked a bit stunned, and immediately started to cry. All the help I had called for now started pouring into the room: residents, nurses, medical students, pediatricians, and an attending physician. I held onto the delivery table for fear I would pass out. My adrenaline rush was so powerful. I was visibly shaking. Ms. T was once again quiet. The flurry of activity began again. All I could think at the moment was, wow, unknown twins, breech vaginal delivery, oh my God, all that paperwork. Welcome to my fourth year.

11

Three's a Dangerous Crowd

During my fourth year of residency, Nurse G was pregnant with triplets. Here was a new opportunity for me to care for a high order multiple pregnancy. In vitro fertilization and many other assisted reproductive practices were not as common as today. Also, I worked in a county facility. We mostly cared for mid-to-lower socioeconomic status patients: those on Medicaid and government assisted health insurance. Unless a woman spontaneously became pregnant with triplets, we rarely saw patients who could afford many of the procedures that would result in a triplet or higher order pregnancy.

Nurse G, however, worked in the hospital. She opted to have her care at our hospital, and to ultimately deliver with us as well. I learned a lot of lessons during her pregnancy: women carrying triplets almost always end up on bedrest by the 28th week; triplets are almost always delivered by 33 to 34 weeks, 35 if they are lucky. Triplets need lots of monitoring. A C section is always recommended because of the possibility of poor positioning and getting entangled during the delivery. Patients are at higher risk for hypertension, diabetes, preterm labor, preterm rupture of membranes, and many other pregnancy complications.

Imagine growing three separate bodies inside of you. I happened to be on call when she came in at 34 weeks in labor, needing to be delivered. The attending physician scrubbed in with me. After four years of C sections as a resident, I was excited to be doing something I had never done before. Three separate teams were assembled in the OR, ready to take care of three premature babies. An excited buzz hummed through Labor and Delivery. The initial preparations were about the same as a regular C section, but after the first cut, nothing was the same. When I surveyed the patient on the operating room table, I was quite amazed at the size of her very pregnant belly. Thirty four weeks with triplets looked like a pregnancy with a giant baby inside. I marveled for about the millionth time during my residency at the body's ability to expand for pregnancy and then later contract.

Once I made the incision into the uterus, and broke the bag of water protecting the first baby, Baby A, everything seemed to move in slow motion and fast forward at the same time. Baby A came out pretty easily, head first, crying. She was handed off to the first set of pediatricians. We then had to quickly identify and move Baby B into position for delivery. My first-assistant pushed gently down on the outside of the belly, to move the baby down. I could then break the second bag of water and deliver the second baby, which I was also able to do, with a bit more difficulty than Baby A. B was whisked away to be examined by the pediatrician on the far side of the room. By this time, Nurse G was bleeding significantly. We needed to move more quickly.

I felt the adrenaline reaction that I had felt so many times in the middle of deliveries or surgeries where my body started responding to the events getting serious. I needed to speed up. The attending once again started pushing on Nurse G's abdomen to try to get the third and last baby into position for delivery. At the same time, I reached my hand up inside the giant uterus that was more like a soft bloody rag than a muscular organ designed to contract to push its contents out. All I could feel were small feet and legs, through the last amniotic sac. The baby's back was down, a back-down-transverse lie. The position makes maneuvering a baby out for delivery difficult as it requires pushing and pulling to get the baby into the right position.

I let go of the feet and pushed the baby back up and toward me to get it into a back up position that would be easier for the delivery. Once I did this, I was again able to grab the feet and this time pull them gently down toward the uterine incision. Then I broke the third amniotic sac. The entire OR remained deadly silent. Once the sac was broken, we could see that the fluid was dark greenish, signifying that the baby had felt stress and had a bowel movement inside the sac, hopefully only fairly recently during the manipulation of the delivery. I pulled the feet and legs through the uterine incision, brought out the hips, and then quite automatically did the maneuvers of a breech delivery: hip, turn, sweep down one arm, turn back, sweep down the other arm, pull the feet straight up, flex the head, and pop the head out of the incision.

Baby C came out lifeless. He didn't move, didn't cry, and didn't seem to have any tone to his tiny body. He was smaller than the other two babies. I speedily cut the umbilical cord, lifted this small rag-doll, and passed him off to the third group of pediatricians for what turned out to be a full resuscitation. Adrenaline was high. I was going as fast as I could to safely clean out the uterus, sew it back together, and order lots of medications to help the uterus contract, all while keeping one ear to the table on my right where they were working on the baby. I was almost to the closure of the skin when I heard a small, weak cry from the direction of the C team. The baby was moving a bit, had a good heart rate, but needed help to breathe. I thought I may need some help to breathe as well by that point, but I finished the C section, and waited to hear what was happening in the NICU, which is where all the babies had been taken by then. We got word that A and B were just fine. C was on oxygen but seemed like he'd be okay. Sweet relief. So many emotions from the first cut to the last stitch.

12

The Happy Specialty Except When It's Not

In the winter of my fourth residency year, I was the Chief Gynecology resident for a three month period. I was in charge of all the surgeries and all the gynecologic care we provided in our clinic and to hospital patients. I had a team of residents, medical students, nurse practitioners, and physicians assistants to supervise and teach. All were tasked with taking care of the women on our service.

One afternoon, we were in the general gynecology clinic, taking care of visits for birth control, infections, and pap smears, when I got a call from the emergency room. The second year resident's job was to evaluate emergency gynecology patients, but if a patient might need surgery, I was consulted. Ms. L had come into the ER with severe abdominal pain. She was actually from out of town, young, recently married, and in New York on her honeymoon. She and her new husband were out to dinner when she suddenly had such severe pain that she nearly passed out. She started throwing up. An ambulance was called. She was in the ER being evaluated by my second year resident. She might be a surgical candidate.

I went down to the ER to see what was what. The list of gynecologic conditions that can cause that scenario is short, but some of them would require surgery. It was also possible that this was not a gynecological problem, in which case we would be turfing the case to a general surgeon or whoever was in charge of the organ needing treatment or removal. That could be urological, gastroenterological, orthopedic, or a number of other specialties.

The assumption was usually that women with abdominal pain had a gynecological condition until proven otherwise. The resident had done a good job of examining and ordering the proper tests. Ms. L looked in moderate distress, in spite of pain medication. Her pregnancy test was negative, essentially ruling out something pregnancy related. Her blood work showed inflammation but not necessarily a severe infection. She didn't have a fever. Cultures from her urine and vagina were negative. She had no medical problems, had never been pregnant and had never had abdominal surgery. This ruled out a whole host of other problems: scar tissue, pelvic infection, or pelvic inflammatory disease. A pelvic sonogram showed a large, leaking, possibly twisted, ovarian cyst.

We had to make a diagnosis. The ER physician and the second year resident agreed. This was likely a twisted large ovarian cyst, which was causing severe acute abdominal pain. The solution would be surgery. We should take her to the OR. We could operate through a laparoscope, a small camera that would be placed through the belly button while the patient was under general anesthesia. This would allow us to look into the pelvic cavity, see up close what the problem was, and then deal with it via small incisions with long instruments. We could then either untwist it, remove the cyst, remove the ovary, and do whatever we needed to do to put this poor patient out of her misery.

I agreed after speaking to the patient, examining her myself, and looking at all the test results. Time was crucial since a twisted ovary and cyst could lose its blood supply. If we waited too long we would not be able to save the ovary. I contacted my attending physician, who needed to supervise all surgeries. He agreed. Orders were written, consents were obtained, her husband was spoken to, and the patient was readied for a surgical procedure. I went to the OR with my second year resident and our entourage of students to await the patient's arrival.

Ms. L was wheeled in on a gurney, already almost half asleep from the pain medication and the anti-anxiety meds that the anesthesiologist had given her on the way up. We got her prepped and draped. We were ready to fix this. Over the past few years I had realized that there was something about surgery that appealed to me. It was often black and white. Here was an ailment, a diseased organ, or something inside the body that was not right. Surgery gave me the ability to remove, fix, or correct what was wrong. Usually, the patient would get better. There was something satisfying about knowing what I expected to find when I looked inside someone's body. I knew what had to be done, and had the skills to do it. I had to distance myself from the fact that I had my hands inside someone's body. I thought of this more as a science project that I had to put together. When the surgery was done, the problem would be fixed. Everything would again work properly. Of course, every once in a while, things didn't work out exactly like that.

Ms. L was one of those times. After preparing this patient for her surgical procedure, and arranging ourselves around the operating room table, I took the place of the primary surgeon with my second year across from me. The attending was scrubbed, but standing a bit off to the side. I infiltrated the area under the belly button with local anesthesia. We lifted the sides of the indented belly button so I could carefully place the first trocar, the sleeve through which the camera would then be placed. We insufflated the abdomen with enough CO_2 gas so that we'd be able to have a clear picture through the camera. We placed the camera, attached to a light source, through the sleeve. We turned our attention to the video screens placed strategically so we could see what we were looking at inside the abdomen.

Once we got a good look, we all gasped. The room got silent. What we saw was a large left sided ovarian tumor. Throughout the entire rest of her abdominal cavity we saw signs of a cancer that had spread onto her intestines, on the outer surface of her uterus, under her diaphragm, on her fallopian tubes. We barely saw any surface in her abdominal cavity that was free of what we could assume was spreading and metastatic ovarian cancer.

As we inspected the area with the camera, the attending and I, who had seen ovarian cancer like this before, were continually gasping at each new surface the camera focused on. The phrase "Oh my God" passed my lips, as I thought of how unusual this was, how young this newlywed was, how serious this was, and how her entire life had just changed in the blink of an eye.

We put a call out to the gynecologic oncologist so he could come to the OR and decide what to do. My attending spoke to me about going out to this woman's husband to tell him what was happening. Now we needed permission we did not have, permission to do much more, more necessary surgery than we had gotten the patient's consent for. I was dreading that conversation as I thought about heading to the family waiting area. How do you tell someone who just got married that his new wife had stage four ovarian cancer?

I waited for the gynecologic oncologist to come into the OR to give his opinion before going out to talk to the husband. I did not know what I was going to tell him yet. The oncologist arrived, scrubbed in, and did his meticulous oncologist-assessment. Looking at her entire abdomen, taking his time, his serious and stern expression never wavering, he finally looked up and said, "Nothing to do."

I wasn't sure I heard him correctly. "Nothing to do"? I thought he would immediately get out his scalpel and begin an extensive debulking surgery to remove whatever tumor was evident in her abdomen. Everyone knew that ovarian cancer, left alone, would kill someone in a relatively short time. It was that kind of cancer. In all I had learned, I knew it wasn't like uterine (endometrial) cancer. You could almost always cure that with surgery or cervical cancer, which was now rare because of Pap smears and treatment of cervical precancerous conditions. Ovarian cancer was almost always discovered in its later stages. Even with treatment most of the time this cancer is a death sentence. I waited for him to continue.

"The disease is just so extensive that surgery is not going to help her. The best we can do is to try some chemotherapy and try to shrink what's already in there. If she survives that, we may be able to operate later on to remove what's left." And that was that.

I tried to wrap my head around that and come up with something that would make any sense to this woman's husband. I knew whatever I said was going to be devastating, life-changing, and not believable. But go find the husband in the lobby I did. When I got there I saw her newly-wed husband, that I recognized from the pre-op area. He waited there back in the time where we thought that Ms. L likely had a run-of-the-mill ruptured ovarian cyst or a torsed ovary. The worst I might have told him was that she had lost an ovary during the surgery. He stood up when he saw me. I looked him right in the eye. I owed him that. I sat down, so he would sit, too. All of this had been rehearsed in my mind on the way down from the OR: sit-when-delivering-bad-news, look right-in-his-eyes.

When the husband saw my face, he knew something was not right. "When we went into the OR, we thought that this was likely an ovarian cyst that was rupturing, or an ovary that was twisting, because these are the most likely things it could have been in someone so young," I began. I was trying to tell the story, soften the blow, have him follow the words that would ultimately come to the conclusion I needed him to hear. I could see him anticipating me telling him just which one of these things it had been.

"But sometimes," I went on, "we go in thinking one thing, but once we get in there, it turns out to be entirely something else." Now I could see that running through his mind were likely things like, "Oh, we thought it was an ovary, but it was really her appendix or her gall bladder. So now you are here to tell me that you were wrong, and you had to take out some other organ."

Before he could express those thoughts, I said, "And sometimes, we are all extremely surprised because we find something that we had hoped it wasn't, something very rare. We found it, and we have to change the plan."

My voice started to fail me at this point. I felt a tear run down my face. I had to stop dancing around, and just say it. The moment had come, and he knew it.

"I am so sorry to have to tell you this. Your wife has ovarian cancer." Then I stopped talking for a moment to let those words sink in. They did. He started to cry. We both just sat there for a few moments.

One thing I actually did not have to figure out — one thing I already knew was that I was in The Happy Specialty. Delivering babies, helping women get pregnant, even operating on people and somehow fixing them — were all reasons for celebration. They are times for smiling, bonding with patients and families, and sharing good news, except when not, except when the news is bad, and there is no celebrating.

When things go wrong, when there are unexpected results or poor outcomes as we describe them in medical terms, things go horribly, terribly wrong. Those times are devastating.

This would not be the last time I would have to break bad news to a family and to a patient. There would be deaths, compromised babies, cancers, and unexpected test results. I had not been great in the past at telling people exactly how it was. I had no training, no role models, and no medical school classes in how to break bad news with empathy and kindness. I would need to make sure they heard the truth. I had to become good at exactly that, saying the truth, for this time and the future when I would inevitably and unfortunately again find myself in a similar situation.

13

Expect the Unexpected

On call had a totally different meaning in the world of private practice. For 24 hours I carried a beeper that could go off any time, summoning me that any number of things could be happening. Often patients were calling with questions, or because they needed a prescription and couldn't wait until the next day when the office opened.

They rarely called with emergencies that needed to be tended to right now. Being new to the world of private patients, I took every call very seriously that came through the answering service and, consequently, to my beeper. If a patient called in the middle of the night and said she had pain, I sent her to the ER to be evaluated. I would meet her there. If a new mom called and said she was bleeding more than normal, I would have her go in to be checked. I would meet her at the hospital. In those first few months of carrying the beeper on call, I was going into the emergency room or the delivery room all the time because I was so afraid to miss something.

Ms. C called the answering service one night, and they paged me. She was explaining her situation to me, pregnant, seven months (32 weeks) and on medication for high blood pressure. She had been told about the warning signs for worsening blood pressure problems, and called because she had a very bad headache that would not go away with rest and Tylenol. I advised her to go into the delivery room to be checked. I got up and ready to go and meet her there. I was always thinking of the worst case scenario, never wanting to miss something that should have been taken care of emergently because I might not have correctly assessed the situation.

I went into the delivery room at one of the small local hospitals. I actually got there before Ms. C. I was sitting at the desk when she walked in. I looked up just in time to see her come through the front door, collapse on the floor, shaking in what looked like a full-blown seizure. I went into auto-mode as I had been taught in my residency. Seizures in pregnancy are a sign of eclampsia until proven otherwise. Eclampsia is the end result of a constellation of things, usually in the third trimester of pregnancy, which includes high blood pressure, headache, swelling, and abnormal liver functions. When the swelling gets to the brain, it causes seizures.

The treatment was to stabilize the patient and deliver the baby. The nurses and I ran over, got her on to a bed, and tried to place an IV. This is quite a feat when someone is seizing. I ordered medication to sedate her and bring her blood pressure down. We listened for a heartbeat on the baby, and heard a slow, but steady rate. I called the anesthesiologist in. We all moved quickly toward the OR and prepared the patient for an emergency C section.

All these things were going on simultaneously. I was about to perform my first truly emergent C section in my new, private practice life. The staff was assembled in the OR. I waited for the signal from the anesthesiologist that the patient was deeply asleep under general anesthesia. I took the knife, and made a larger-than-normal transverse incision in the lower abdomen, and proceeded from there, with all the sharp instruments and my hands. There was so much bleeding because a person with eclampsia does not have blood that clots normally. I moved as fast as I could to reach the uterus, and finally the baby. He was out in two minutes and was tiny but crying. I handed him to the pediatric staff waiting by the warmer.

Once the baby was out, the entire room breathed a collective sigh of relief, and we began the closure. The bleeding was eventually controlled. Ms. C went to the ICU, still intubated, on a respirator. She and the baby had a long road ahead.

I was so relieved that I had done my residency in a place where I had seen this exact scenario more than once. I was ready to handle it. And I was elated that I had taken my beeper so seriously.

14

A Routine Delivery, Except When Not

One Saturday I was on call as an attending physician. A patient pregnant with her second baby called the answering service. Ms. Q was 38 weeks along. I had seen her pretty regularly throughout her pregnancy, which was generally uncomplicated. She and I had formed a bond. She had made most of her prenatal appointments with me. When the answering service contacted me, I called her back. Ms. Q told me she thought, "This was it." She thought she was in enough labor to go to the hospital.

The usual procedure was she would go to the hospital, a nurse in Labor and Delivery would examine her and then call me. When the patient was in active labor, I would go in, and manage the advanced stages of her labor until delivery, whenever that would be. Uncomplicated multips, or patients that had already had one or more successful deliveries, were my favorite. They were likely to have another successful and uncomplicated vaginal delivery, but not always. Once I had someone that was admitted in labor, I would arrange my subsequent hours of the day, assuming I'd shortly be going into the hospital, only to return home after the delivery was complete.

The nurse called me with an assessment, "The patient is uncomfortable, contracting every three minutes. She is three to four centimeters dilated. The baby looks reassuring on the monitor. Water's not broken."

That assessment told me for someone having her second baby, it would likely not be long until she was in active labor. I asked the nurse a few questions. All seemed well. Ms. Q wanted an epidural, since she was getting more uncomfortable pretty quickly, and had had one during her first delivery. She felt it had helped her get through her active phase of labor. I recommended that the patient get the epidural soon, and started making my way over to the hospital. When I got to the hospital, I felt the timing was great. Ms. Q had gotten her epidural, was quite comfortable, and glad to see me.

We talked for a few moments, and I asked her all of the usual admission questions. Although she was not feeling pain, I could tell from the monitor that she was having strong, frequent, and regular contractions. I asked if she wanted me to recheck her cervix since it had now been several hours since she arrived. She said yes. I put on gloves for the exam. I was still in my street clothes, as I usually changed into scrubs closer to the time the delivery was imminent. When I examined her, I remember thinking, "This is good" because her cervix was 5 centimeters dilated, and the head felt well-applied to the cervix. There was a fairly large "bag of water"— the amniotic sac, which I was able to feel in front of the baby's head. I advised that I could break the bag of water. The contractions would likely get stronger, moving along toward her delivery. Ms. Q agreed.

We have a little device, a plastic hook that we use to poke the amniotic sac so it breaks. I always followed the rules when it came to breaking waters during labor — never too early, never when the head is not well-applied to the cervix. In this case, it felt like I was again following the rules. However, in labor, as in life, anything can happen. It sure did here. I poked the sac gently with my plastic hook, and instead of the baby's head moving further down towards delivery, I immediately felt a soft, spongy, pulsing piece of tissue. It took me about 3 seconds to realize that this was the baby's umbilical cord, creating what is called a prolapsed cord, and is a life-threatening emergency for the baby. If part of the umbilical cord comes out, and if it cannot be pushed back up inside the uterus, it will be compressed, cutting off the blood flow to the baby that has been keeping it alive.

This is one of those things that causes an automatic reaction in any birth attendant that has ever had the misfortune to have seen this before. During my residency, I had seen it twice. The auto-response is to call out that the cord has prolapsed, and that we need a stat C section. This is one of those rare times that the current situation does mimic a medical TV show with people yelling "STAT" and running around, getting things ready, grabbing instruments, and seeming like a disorganized fire drill.

I tried to push the umbilical cord back up inside as firmly as I could, trying to get it up behind the baby's head.

This was almost impossible, now that the head was tightly against the cervix, blocking me from getting around it to move the cord back up and relieve the pressure. I climbed up on the labor bed with the patient, and tried to hold the cord up there, attempting to move the baby's head up and away from the cord as best as I could. I watched the fetal heart rate monitor, which was starting to signal distress. I was loudly giving orders for the nurses to push the labor bed immediately back to the OR with me still in my street clothes on it with the patient, trying at the same time not to scare the patient. Pretty impossible. All of this happened in a matter of five very long minutes.

We were quickly back in the OR. Nurses were cleaning her belly, calling other doctors, grabbing instruments, and covering me and the patient with drapes. The anesthesiologist quickly put the patient under general anesthesia, and said, "GO". I grabbed the knife and did the fastest incision I had ever made, ignoring the blood and the cosmetic effect. The baby was out within minutes. By that time there were two other doctors in the OR. I left the room to wash and change my clothes, noting that the baby was being evaluated by the pediatricians on my way out. By the time I came back into the OR, the baby was crying and things were much calmer. I scrubbed, gowned, and gloved, and finished the C section, assisted by one of the other doctors. Only after everything was done was I able to step back, take a deep breath, and think about what had happened.

From the moment I had realized the emergent nature of the situation, until the end of the C section, all of 20 minutes had passed. Yet the time seemed like hours and moments all at the same time. Having encountered this situation before created an automatic set of actions where I simultaneously assessed and directed the situation. Only when I finally had the time to look back on what had happened did I fully realize how tragic the outcome could have been. Babies cannot live without constant flow through their umbilical cord for longer than a few moments without dire consequences. Pushing a patient's bed to the OR with a physician practically on top of the patient, with one hand in the vagina, pushing the umbilical cord up, and doing a one-handed cesarean section while still in street clothes is what had to be done to result in a live and non-compromised baby. So that is just what I did.

15

My Upside Down Night
with a Butt-Side Down Baby

One night I was on call as an attending physician. Ms. B called and said she felt like she was going into labor. I didn't recognize her name. That wasn't too unusual because I practiced in a group of physicians. Ms. B had possibly seen the other providers for her prenatal visits. I had a pretty good memory for patients in the practice who were close to delivering. When she told me she was getting uncomfortable, I recommended she go to the hospital. I would meet her there.

At that time, all records were on paper. Periodically during a pregnancy we would fax those records to the delivery room so we and the hospital would have the medical and prenatal history of each patient coming in for delivery. I called the hospital delivery room to let them know Ms. B was on her way. I was surprised when the nurse said they didn't have a copy of her prenatal records on file. This rarely happened, and was one of my most unfavorite occurrences for my on call nights. That meant trekking to my office at night, going through our filing cabinet of prenatal records, faxing or making a copy, and bringing the copy with me to the hospital. When I think of how inefficient and antiquated that system was, I cringe. Now we just go onto any computer and pull up any patient's prenatal record from our electronic record website.

I went to my office, dug into our prenatal filing cabinet. I then realized why I hadn't recognized her name, and didn't know her history. Her prenatal record had exactly one visit. Ms. B had come into our office to confirm her pregnancy. We had made several other appointments, which she always cancelled or rescheduled, and then failed to show up. A failure of our system was not having an alarm system to tell us when a patient, especially a pregnant patient, did not show up for visits. No one had caught the no-shows or the re-schedules. No one had expected her to show up in labor, since no one knew her. Now that I took her phone call and now that no one had ever formally discharged her from our practice, I had no choice but to meet her at the hospital. She still had a relationship with our practice even though she hadn't come in for any of her other prenatal visits. Medical liability is strange that way.

When I got to the hospital, with my less-than-one-page prenatal chart, I understood a little more. I was in Labor and Delivery, but the patient wasn't yet there. Ms. B had called me and said she would go to the hospital. I had first gone all the way to my office and then to the hospital. She still wasn't there. That made me suspect that she might not show up at all. I called the phone number listed on the prenatal record, such as it was, not really a record, and got an answering machine.

Now I had a dilemma: Do I assume she is coming and wait? And then deliver someone I don't at all know, taking on the liability of this delivery of someone who has been completely non-compliant with her prenatal care? I didn't have time to contemplate. While I was discussing my concerns with the delivery room nurse, the doors to the delivery room suddenly opened. A couple walked in, the man in his 30s, looking scared, and the woman, obviously in her third trimester of pregnancy, bent over and screaming in pain, the type of pain I had seen so many times before when a laboring woman was going through transition with no pain medication. Screaming and breathing, holding her belly, writhing in pain, and then quiet for a few moments until the next contraction hit, then repeat the whole scenario but louder.

We took under ten seconds to move into action. The nurses ran over with a wheelchair. When the screaming, laboring woman sat down, I could see the thing that makes us all breathe hard and move even faster, a thick stream of green fluid pouring down her inner thighs, meconium, a sign of fetal distress while a baby is still in utero. Meconium usually means the baby would need to come out soon. From the look of the pregnant woman, the baby would likely be coming out very soon anyway. The nurses and I leapt into action, asking questions, putting on monitors, pulling out IV bags and tubing from the supply shelves. Ms. B spoke in spurts between her contractions.

Her story went like this: This was her first pregnancy, first baby, and she had come to our office once, to verify her pregnancy. Her due date was about a week ago. She had been in the care of a home-birth midwife who was planning to deliver the baby at her home, in a birthing tub. Ms. B had not had any ultrasounds or lab work. "Unnecessary interventions," according to her midwife. Ms. B had spent the last two days laboring at home, waiting. Her water had broken about 12 hours ago. She had continued to have amniotic fluid leakage that went initially from clear, to bloody, to what was now an obviously brownish-green color that was getting progressively thicker.

Her home-birth midwife was apparently unconcerned. In the last few hours, Ms. B and her husband decided the pain was too great. They started to get worried and to doubt the midwife. They called our answering service to have me deliver her at the hospital. Wow. So much information, but no time to review it all in my head. Only time to act.

Ms. B did not want to stay seated. She did not want to stay lying down. She wanted to be standing up and rocking and screaming. It was impossible for me to examine her without her staying in one place. Although it is totally out of character for me to raise my voice while a patient is in labor, this time I did. I implored her to get onto the bed just for a moment so I could at least check her cervix to see if she could push. She ignored me, continuing to scream, holding onto her significant other, and rocking back and forth. Even between contractions she couldn't stay still.

I did the only thing I could with her standing and rocking. I put on my gloves, and knelt down on the floor under her. From that incredibly awkward, upside-down position I attempted to do a vaginal exam. I almost passed out when I examined and found her cervix was not completely dilated, and her baby's butt, with meconium streaming out of it, was right at the opening to the cervix.

Not only that. A pair of swollen, bluish testicles were hanging just below the not-completely-dilated cervix. Apparently, her home-birth midwife did not realize what she was feeling as the patient became more and more dilated. Then it became apparent that this was not the baby's head. Maybe they had better get over to the hospital for management. I immediately called out, "Open the OR" to get everyone ready for an emergent C section. A flurry of activity began, calling the anesthesiologist, scrubbing the room, getting out instruments.

I looked at the patient and said, "You need to have a C section right now!" in my sternest-trying-not-to-freak-her-out voice. As I was saying this, I was following the usual protocol to get ready for a C section: ask her many pertinent questions, describe the procedure to get her informed consent, explain the situation, breech baby, already in distress, and a week past the due date, with an incompletely dilated cervix. Before I was even finished with my explanation, she held up her hand as if to signal me to stop talking. "No," she said, "I'm not having a C section!"

I don't know if I have ever said these words before or since that day. I looked her straight in the eye and said, "If you don't have a C section, your baby's testicles are going to fall off!" This was the truth.

I was only imagining at that point all the worrisome things that could have been going on with her baby. It was breech, and was releasing dark thick meconium, a sign of distress. The meconium was trailing down her legs, and continuous. The testicles were already swollen and blue. It wouldn't be long before they lost all their blood supply. Who knows where the umbilical cord was or how the baby's heart rate had been over the last minutes or hours that her labor was going on? This baby needed to come out now. Of course, it is impossible and illegal to take someone to a surgery that they are refusing to have, unless they are somehow incapable of making that decision. While I thought she was acting crazy, she clearly knew what I was saying. Time was running out for the poor baby.

In my four years of residency, and what was now two or so years as an attending, I had seen plenty of patients who said they didn't want a C section. I even had a few who said they wouldn't consent to one, but then changed their minds given worrisome circumstances. I had never had one that had outright refused when faced with the possibility that the baby would be damaged, or possibly not survive if she didn't agree. And now, here we were. Ms. B was tied to the idea that her birth would be "all natural," and her body was "meant to give birth." She believed that was the only way she could give birth. She believed she was getting proper and wonderful care from her home-birth midwife.

The reality was that the midwife was leading her astray. Her midwife could not even tell that the baby was not in a head down position, and that these were testicles, swollen and blue, that were trying to be delivered first. The patient had not even considered the idea that the baby would be delivered any way but vaginally in her own home surrounded by friends and family with mood lighting and incense. She hadn't gotten the usual educational visits that we typically had with patients. She hadn't had ultrasounds. All the standard discussions never took place. Now I was asking her to trust me when she didn't even know me. She continued to stand holding onto her petrified-looking partner, who was trying to be supportive of her.

I tried in my best "We don't-have-a-lot-of-time-to-decide" voice to approach this from all angles. I told them I had kids. I told them that I had given birth twice, and things don't always work out the way we plan. I told them I would do anything to protect and save my children from pain and damage. I told them I had seen this once before and the testicles had to be amputated. Yes, I used that word. The testicles lost their blood supply and couldn't be saved. This wasn't really a part of my experience, but I had read about a case like that. I told them that if we went to the OR right now, she may still be able to be awake for the surgery instead of being put under general anesthesia. We were running out of time. I think the idea that the testicles may not survive finally hit a nerve with her partner, maybe empathy pains. He was convincing her to listen to me.

Ms. B looked terrified and exhausted. She gave up. She allowed us to gently lift her up onto a gurney. We wheeled her into the OR. The anesthesiologist was standing by and the OR was ready and waiting. I listened to the baby's heartbeat, noting that we still had a little time. I tried to explain everything that was happening, the need to lie this way, move that way, so the anesthesiologist could quickly get the spinal anesthetic into her. He gave her anti-anxiety medication through the swiftly placed IV.

I started the surgery. About three minutes later, when I extracted the baby through the C section scar, I noted the extremely swollen and blue testicles and immediately handed the baby off to the pediatrician in the delivery room. I finished up what was ultimately a bloodier-than-usual C section, but not much different than many stat C sections I had already done.

I tried to be reassuring. Ms. B was awake and mostly alert. Her partner was sitting next to her head, trying to watch everything that was going on. I had no idea how her baby was faring until we were all done, and the pediatrician came in to speak with them. He told them it seemed that the baby and his testicles were probably going to be fine. Had it been just a few more moments, then they might not have been able to save the testicles since the blood supply was so severely compromised for so long.

I wasn't sure if Ms. B and her partner were comprehending exactly what the pediatrician was saying. They had had a long, scary few days. Her labor and delivery turned out to be nothing like she had imagined, how they had envisioned it would be. Ms. B's unwillingness to consider any other possible scenarios had almost cost her baby dearly. I promised myself on that day and many times since then that my job, my responsibility, was to educate my patients, to educate pregnant women, about the need for flexibility in their birth plans. They needed to know that there is never just one acceptable scenario for labor and the delivery of their baby. We cannot always control how a baby ultimately enters the world. I have been amazed at how often since then I have had to repeat that same mantra to patients and to myself.

Afterword

There were times during my 20 plus years in obstetrics and gynecology I thought I could not continue. Times when I was awake for three days in a row, when I had to disappoint my family by missing my daughter's vocal concert or my son's baseball game. Sometimes a bad outcome made me question my choices and skill. I would then realize that there could be no other career, no other specialty that would have made me as happy and as fulfilled as this one. No words can describe the feeling of delivering a healthy baby, solving a woman's long-term reproductive problems, or hearing a heart-felt thank you after spending time and effort to ensure a patient feels better.

These stories are a sample of the many episodes that have shaped the story of my life as a practicing physician. Other memories are waiting to be put to paper.

To be continued.

Thank You

To my colleagues, mentors, and fellow physicians. These stories have more of your input than you know. Thank you to the Labor and Delivery nurses and midwives I have had the privilege to work with through the years. You have shown me special ways to care for women having babies.

Individual heartfelt thanks to some extraordinary people:

My dear friend Patti — for always listening and giving me advice, even when I wouldn't listen.

Dr. Tom Erhardt — for calling me when a residency spot opened up, which changed my life.

Dr. Cheryl Solomon — (RIP) for teaching me a surgical technique I still use 25 years later. Chapter 6 is for you.

Dr. Nick Khulpateea — for showing me the beauty of practically bloodless surgery, and for introducing me to your wife, Taru.

Dr. Taru Khulpateea — for taking a chance and hiring me right out of residency.

Dr. Jerome Solomon — for hiring me when I moved across the country and making me feel welcome in your California practice.

To the wonderful women at my practice, Premier ObGyn Napa Inc., who have helped me open and run a successful solo private practice in difficult, trying times.

To my stepsons, **Carson and Alex** — for welcoming me into your family even when I was monopolizing your dad.

To my children, **Jacob, Danielle, and Dylan** — I love you more than words can say. Thank you for supporting me in this journey, even when I know it wasn't always easy for you and when I talked about placentas at the dinner table.

And of course, to my amazing husband, **Bill** — my rock, my source of strength whether I come home laughing or in tears, my partner in travel and in life — I dedicate this book to you.

CPSIA information can be obtained
at www.ICGtesting.com
Printed in the USA
BVHW040807250420
578457BV00014B/3101

9 781941 066416